The really, really, really, useful guide
Number 13

Go

Fat

Go

MIKE PEARCE

Copyright 2018 by Mike Pearce

All rights reserved. No part of this book may be reproduced, distributed or transmitted in any form or by any means, including photocopying, recording, or other electronic or mechanical methods, without the prior written permission of the author, except in the case of brief quotations embodied in reviews and certain other non-commercial uses permitted by copyright law. You must not circulate this book in any format.

This book may not be resold or given away to other people. Please respect the work of the author and purchase a copy for you own use.

This is a fictional work and all characters are drawn from the author's imagination. Any resemblance or similarities to persons living or dead are entirely coincidental

ISBN:10-1721917551
ISBN-13:978-1721917556

DEDICATION

This book is dedicated to all those worrying about their
weight and would like to change their lives by losing even a
few pounds

CONTENTS

ACKNOWLEDGMENTS

The author would like to thank Christine Pearce
for reading and checking through the manuscript.

PREFACE

It is always easier to gain calories than lose them. Many people today are hugely overweight. Society is accepting them as a new norm whereas in the past they could have been exhibited in a Barnham like sideshow. With this increase in size can come serious health problems.

Eating for some is just emotional hunger, a habit not a necessity. Breaking this cycle and through repetition of new habits one can create spectacularly changes in one's health and lifestyle. Don't end up as a lethargic, inactive, bloated mass, full of wind on a downward spiral towards a serious health disorder and certain death. This book outlines why we want to lose weight, why to some people big is beautiful and the concern of many with butt size.

1 REASONS FOR LOSING WEIGHT

There are many reasons for wanting to lose weight. The major one is because of health problems being threat of heart disease, stroke, stress on joints such as knee and arthritis. Heavy people may experience pain in the chest mistaken for a heart attack which brings on worry. There has been a massive increase in diabetes type 2 and in extreme cases this has meant loss of toes or even limbs. However losing weight can sometimes reverse diabetes type 2 and will make you feel better by increasing endorphins which give the feel-good factor. One can feel fitter and healthier. The stress of just managing day to day can disappear.

Heavy people may become tired when walking or climbing the stairs. They may not be able to play ball games with their children or sit on rides in the amusement park. Also, they are restless and don't sleep well at night. A good sleep is needed to prevent craving for more energy foods. When lying down fat can block airways causing difficulty in breathing.

Where there are larger folds of skin you may produce much more sweat and retain heat in these areas encouraging fungal infections. Losing weight can result in lifestyle changes giving you a complete change of outlook on life, increased confidence, and a change in mood.

The image in society of overweight, heavy children and adults is common place. These are often ridiculed, stigmatised, criticised, abused and made fun of. This links back with times when fat ladies were put in freak shows and people paid money to see them. Putting on weight can encourage guilt and often creates fear of what friends may say behind your back or whether you are being rejected by their partner because you've changed. Also, being fat with a food baby may make people think you are pregnant. They may even congratulate you and embarrass you when they ask to touch your bump!

Often being overweight makes you unhappy, especially if you become unable to fit comfortably into clothes and cannot portray a slim look. The need to be able to fit comfortably into seats, go onto the beach or sit around a swimming pool in a bikini and possibly attract the opposite sex is unfulfilled. Some women slim so that they will look fantastic in a wedding dress or just presentable at a job interview. This must not be the final goal as after the wedding their determination to lose weight may be lost. To cover up their shape fatter people often have to wear loose, shapeless sack like clothes so as to hide their figure. Others may buy or recycle their smaller size clothes and use them as a target for further weight loss.

Everyone wants to look younger and have thin children. The media and businesses promote slim women and muscular men. They are often seen in successful models and famous icons.

Doctors often fear to label their patients as fat or obese and certainly do not use these words in front of them.

2 LOSING WEIGHT

There are hundreds, possibly thousands of different ways of dieting and losing weight. Often lists are given of foods which you can eat as much as you like and not put on weight. These act as fillers giving the full sensation but not the calories. But unlike animals who are satisfied by just eating grass, humans need to make these foods more attractive and taste good. Often hunger can be linked to thirst and staved off by drinking water.

A lot of the cheapest food found in the shops is the unhealthiest. Diet drinks may not be diet and they give no energy so that you may feel even hungrier. Increased health increases the ability to exercise and strengthen muscles through movement. Inactivity will not burn calories and is a killer. Exercising different muscles will build up a better shape for your body able to withstand anything life can throw at you. Weight loss also gives a boost to the immune system and a trigger for the body to increase its metabolism and burn off fat. To be successful in losing weight one has to form a new state of mind on how one thinks about food and especially overcome past habits and learn to ignore temptations. When one strays from the ideal diet, especially at social events, or eating out with the kids one can develop a sense of guilt. Eat before going to a buffet so that hunger will not force you to eat more. There is a stigma about your weight especially if you feel you are the fattest person in a team or a group. You begin to make excuses and blame events and people that disrupt your efforts to change your eating habits. But you can always compensate for this.

People wanting to lose weight need to get into the better life groove like a needle on an old 78rpm record which kept it in its plastic groove for the whole record, which is the rest of your life. It is easy though to knock one out of the groove, but one still can carry on with the slimming music in another groove.

You need to see what works well. Many slimming organisations have different incentives for keeping people in the groove. These can include certificates, stars, fridge magnets, prizes and praise in front of local groups. One group gives a small jewelled stone for every stone lost. It is imperative to remove the feeling that dieting is pointless if one week you do not lose any weight or put some on by eating non-slimming foods. You have to realise that different people lose weight in diverse ways be it fast or slow. No one can lose a huge amount of weight in one week except by starvation. Some weeks you may not lose any weight at all.

Metabolism can be greater in fatter people as well as energy needs to keep the body ticking over. It is good to buddy up with someone who is also trying to lose weight and can offer some competition. You have faced challenging times before and got over them. Never be discouraged. As long as you make an effort to make these new foods attractive and achieve smaller goals and are satisfied with these certain foods you cannot go wrong. Your body will soon adapt and learn to function on different diets and routines. Your attempts to lose weight can filter down to friends and even your family. It is important not to pander to children's love of fast or fattening foods. Some people think children are little men and should have substantial portions like their fathers. The largest 30 stone, 11-year-old boy was known to have an insatiable appetite and was constantly fed by his mother who kept feeding him because she loved him. Part of the problem also here was his celebrity status which provided an extra income for a poor family. There are plenty of people around who love to encourage you to over eat so beware.

3 BIG IS BEAUTIFUL?

There is no reason to think that big is not beautiful. Big definitely is beautiful in some societies or for some people. Venus figures from the Palaeolithic in Europe, as well as many Greek and Roman statues, emphasised the shape and beauty of the buttocks. In China buttocks are compared to the full moon. Prominent buttocks were common in Hottentots, in some Hispanic and African Americans and established as a norm. Butts have helped humans with balance in a bipedal posture. Big butts are also useful for balancing the weight when pregnant so as to reduce back problems. There is no guarantee that exercise and diet will reduce butt size. Fat may be taken from other parts of the body making the buttocks stand out even more.

Bushmen in the Kalahari Desert can have big buttocks. Large buttocks and hips on Asian, European and African women are seen as a form of beauty. On the other hand, some Japanese regard small hips as beautiful and women often prefer men with small buttocks. Many painters e.g. Rubens, Cezanne and Velasquez emphasise the beauty of large naked bottoms in their pictures. Cherubs in paintings or sculpture are often fat which was seen as a sign of happiness and health. Some women like the excess fat on men's sides and say that these are love handles to hold onto. The size of your butt, whether small or large, can affect self-confidence.

Some women want to increase the size of their butts through exercise and high protein diets. Eating more fat does not make them fatter. In some countries bottoms are spanked or pinched in a friendly way. Today doctors can be in trouble from butt smacking patients whereas in Victorian times it may have been common. Streakers or mooners exposing their bottoms in public to some though may seem abhorrent. A lot of fat on a bottom also in the past helped reduce the pain caused by caning which was used as a punishment for school children or sailors. So why worry about your butt size?

4 WHAT IS A BUTT?

In humans, the largest muscle in the butt is the gluteus maximus. It helps with maintaining our position as well as leg extension when walking, climbing or running. Some countries like Brazil and China have competitions for beautiful bottoms where they wiggle in front of an audience. The shape of one's pelvis is linked to the amount of fat in the buttocks which is thought to indicate the reproductive capability of the person. With more mass on the buttocks the curvature of the back is emphasized which makes women more attractive. One can also wear high heels which helps you push in your chest and thrust your butt backwards.

The gluteus maximus muscles form a crack in the centre which is wider in women so that more of the fat can wiggle. Numerous humorous songs exist which refer to wiggle or shaking. Women also when walking, move their anterior acetabulum, so they swing their hips forward and inward. Elvis being a man, in order to wiggle had to move his hips. There are other animals that have pretty sizable butt cracks such as rhinos and hippos. Chimps and gorillas have a smaller gluteus maximus than humans and do not have human butt sized cracks.

5 BUTTS-ALL CHANGE

The size or shape of the butt can change. During pregnancy the butt size increases and after birth it can take several months to return to its normal size. Weight can also increase after the menopause as your metabolism of fat can slow down. As women age their hourglass figure disappears and their buttocks become like mens. The ligaments lose elasticity with age and drooping occurs. Less oestrogen causes sagging. This encourages fat deposition while testosterone discourages storage.

With life style changes you can get problems. Sitting in a chair for extended periods can cause the gluteal muscles can atrophy. Larger butts can have pressure sores if in lying in bed or sitting in a chair for extended periods. Cycling can help tone your gluteal muscles, especially on the downward thrust and cycling up hills. Other sports such as swimming, running and football can also help. Kickbacks, step ups, squats and lunges forward on one knee are often recommended in exercise sessions to strengthen the butt.

Bottoms can vary in shape, but you need to realise that the yellow fat in your butt is not dangerous like body fat. Fat in the butt rather than on the belly is better for you as it has less effect on the body's organs. The H shaped bottom is straight up and down below the waist; square- with prominent hip bones rather like a man. This body type contains low amounts of fat at their waist.

Other people have a round cherry like bottom. Here the fat is on the upper cheeks. The main problem with this cherry shape is that there is too much fat in the butt which can make this butt disproportionate to the rest of the body.

Those people with a V shape bottom have fullness at the hips and top of the butt, but narrow in size and shape towards the bottom of the butt

There is also the Inverted "V"-Shaped Butt: Here the waist is smaller than the hips and the butt is much bigger than the waist.

The butt which is sometimes thought the most attractive is the heart or pear shaped like an upside-down heart.

You can't really make an enormous difference to the size of the butt without plastic surgery. Pockets of fat can be removed from buttocks using cannulas less than 3mm diameter. Tiny incisions are made for liposuction. No more than 40% should be removed or it can look saggy or the skin wrinkles. You can have a butt lift where excess fat is removed from the sagging bottom and the skin is pulled up.

To increase the size of the butt one can't inject fat into the buttocks as it is reabsorbed by the body. Butt implants involve injecting silica through incisions made between the muscle and fat. However, injections of silica can be dangerous. It is difficult to try to remodel the H shaped bottom. The heart shaped butt is easy to remodel but there is not a lot of fat to relocate. Sometimes the silica can shift causing asymmetrical buttocks.

6 MAKING BUTTS ATTRACTIVE

Male baboons have bright red buttocks and mandrills have bright blue ones to attract females or to indicate aggression. Female apes increase the size of their bottoms when ovulating. High oestrogen levels of the female's hormone produces a prominent bottom.

Bottoms can vary in hairiness. Some apes have large ischial callosities (butt tumours, callused skin) on their bottoms. This prevents injury when falling but their sense organs still feel pain. They are useful to apes if sitting down on hot ground. We don't need these callosities as we have muscles used for cushioning and padding

Some Oklahoma lambs have a mutation that produces large muscular rumps. The mutation is caused 'callpyge,' Greek for beautiful bottom, but the meat is not tender

Bombardier ground beetles spray the unsuspected attacker with a boiling jet of a hot 100-degree centigrade through their bottoms. The mixture of caustic chemicals is held in the abdominal chambers.

In the past hoops, bustles or corsets were worn which helped to push out the buttocks. Corsets often when tight laced in the 19th century squeezed too tight so that only part of the lungs was used for breathing and mucus built up. Corsets in the fifties would help redistribute the fat and minimised the size of the hips. Today tight clothing and high heels exaggerate the buttocks. Padding or moulded panties can be used to try and alter the shape. Some jeans have enhancers attached inside them or one can invest in yoga pants which cover up imperfections. It is believed that dark jeans make the butt look smaller whereas white ones make it look bigger. Wearing trousers with large pockets also make it look smaller but small raised pockets make it look bigger

To make butts more attractive humans can have a tattoo but being in such a position means it is difficult to appreciate it yourself. It is often placed above the trouser line for all to see. Tattoos on the butt can hurt but less so in men. Small or large areas can be tattooed. Letters are popular and large dream catchers.

One can even get buttocks branded. There are fewer nerves in the butt, so it hurts less. Scars heal in three weeks. Ruby or other precious stones can also be attached to the butt. Fortunately, we do not need tails although some people do have soft, boneless, non-functional ones. We no longer have to use them for balance to swish away flies, to grasp branches or to signal to the opposite sex.

Accumulation of fat does have its benefits in body reserves when ill or hungry or abandoned on a desert island. It helps one survive longer and float better in water. It provides food for the unborn and suckling babies. It also cushions our falls and can protect our organs as well as generate many of the chemicals and hormones needed by us to function.

Remember, no matter how fat you are, someone will always love you. Loss of weight needs many little goals to lose weight in small stages. To get a real idea of a small loss in weight try lifting a 2 kg (only 4.4lbs) in one hand and you will realise what you have been carrying round in the past. Destroy your addiction to feel good foods which are bad for you. Change your emotional eating habits where you continually snack just as a habit or to pass the time or help solve a problem. Many believe turning to chocolate or drink will make you better. Possibly initially but it will not last. Don't allow yourself to reach a point where you have one foot in the grave and the other on a banana. Start dieting today.

To see other publications below by the author visit
snappysnappybooks.com

<u>The really, really, really useful series</u>

How to be a Successful Business Weed
How to Deal with Life's Snakes and Ladders
Know Your Students and Build Your Image
Pens for Pops
How to be a Successful Charity Shop
Make up-revealed
Ronnie's Sermon snippets
Wastefulness-Bone and Urine
Fertility Stones and Chocolate Eggs
Clingers, creepers and scramblers
I Herring Gull
Viking Bay-Natural History

<u>Other books by Mike Pearce:</u>

Pattern for Purpose- God's and Man's designs
Red Fred Cell and Friends
Human Termites eat London
Pigeons Splat London
Glass Anemones Tentacle-ize London
Tuppeny Hangover
I am Termite
The littlest Oyster
Bits and Bobs
The Shell Man
Cats at Christmas
Tails, Tales
Trust-Nothing but a Must
In a Dark, Dark Corner was the Holy Ghost
The Shell Lady
Captain Grottbuster versus the Grey World

London's Nemesis (Trilogy of 3, 4 and 5 above
Saved by Angels (Trilogy of 6, 8 and 14 above)
The World of Wax
Photosynthetic Women
Queen Rat on Deadman's Island
The Watcher on the Fal
The Rock Pool
The Little Shepherd Boy's Gift
The Living Fossils
Old Mother Nature Laughed and Laughed
Betty's Barcodes
Time Runs Dry (play)
Valentines Cards
The Scrofula Infirmary
The Cornish Urchin
My Therizinosaurus
Spider in the Tomb
The White Cockerel
The Red Church Doll
Butterfly Angels (compilation of previous books)
The Girl Under the Paeony Tree
Baby Feet
The Sparrows' Last Soul
Ball Rooms
Absorbed by a Woman
St Mildred-Patron Saint of Thanet
The Slothful Wife
The Tuppeny Bear
The Boy who found Christmas
Nothing but leaves
The Giant's Toothpick
The Night Mare
The Old Pot and the Golden Shoes
Sitting next to Angels

Exodus to a leaf
The forlorn fruit fly
The Pawnbroker's Souls
The Nursery Rhyme Cat
A Call Under the Sea
Dead Donkey Lane
A Googolplex of Mice
The Eggstraordinary Easter Egg
The China Blackbird
A slice of Slang with a touch of Cockney and a
drop of Dorset
The Rusty Gate
Beware of Cucumbers, apples and pigs
The Lady loves Red
The woman who smelled books
Till my lips were salt as brine

ABOUT THE AUTHOR

Dr Mike Pearce is a scientist interested in behaviour. He also was a lecturer in human biology and health at a college in Canterbury, Kent